# BEHIND THE SCENES
# OF CANCER
## FOR A LONGER SURVIVAL
## AND BETTER QUALITY OF LIFE

*Maria do Carmo Vieira-Montfils*

# Behind the Scenes of Cancer
## For a longer survival and better quality of life

1st Edition
POD

KBR
Petrópolis
2015

Publisher **Noga Sklar**
Text Edition **KBR**
Cover design **KBR**
Cover Illustration **"Treatment of cancer",
Edo Period, Japan, 1809**

ISBN 978-85-8180-377-7

KBR Editora Digital Ltda.
www.kbrdigital.com
www.facebook.com/kbrdigital
contact@kbrdigital.com
1|864|373.4528

HEA039030 - Health/ Cancer

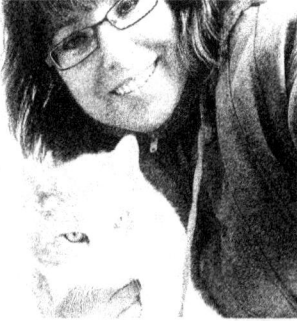

**Maria do Carmo Vieira-Montfils** is a Canadian writer, born in Brazil. She has been living in Canada for 15 years. She had published two books in French, *Fenêtre Virtuelle* (poems) and *Une deuxième vie - aide à la francisation*. *Behind the Scenes of Cancer* is her first book published by KBR, in three languages, Portuguese, French and English. Maria do Carmo is a columnist and a regular contributor to KBR's weekly magazine, *Singles K*.

**E-mail:** maviemontfils@yahoo.ca

# Table of Contents

*In honor of my patients.*

*In gratitude to the doctor and friend who took care of my sister, Wagner Brant Moreira M.D.*

# INTRODUCTION

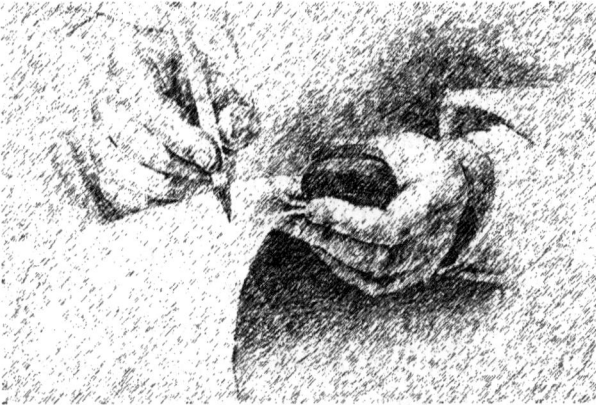

This book is not a document of a professional nature. Due to its informal style, my text resembles an essay and fits very well into my purpose because in this way we can express our ideas and opinions subjectively, with no so many limitations. We do not need to prove anything. At the same time, as I attempt to analyze some points of view and propose a conclusion about the subject, I will make room for a few ethical and philosophical reflections.

Nevertheless, I would not dare to establish any rule.

This is the testimony of a person who lived for a long time in the oncology environment. Despite everything I have learned as an oncologist, I will not give advice or suggestions as a doctor. It is no more than a logical view, above all an attempt to help the smooth flow of human intercourse; furthermore, why not give a hand to science?

It is also my intent to offer new ideas for cancer treatment and to invite everyone to add their contribution to a new approach.

In this way, this essay speaks directly to the patients and those around them — to the health care team, the researcher and others who may possibly be interested in the subject "cancer", keeping an open mind as generous as possible as they meditate about our questions and needs.

I will try to follow with every step we encounter when this disease enters our lives, to establish a way of improving our path, on both sides, that of the patient and that of the healthcare team. Another goal is to search for the right direction for each one, in order to pursue a future where hope is more likely to become a reality.

As the questions I discuss in this book are universal, they might be of interest to everyone, no matter where it is published.

This book is not intended as a substitute for the medical advice of physicians. The reader should regularly consult a physician in matters relating to his or her health and particularly with respect to any symptoms that may require diagnosis or medical attention.

# 1. WHY?

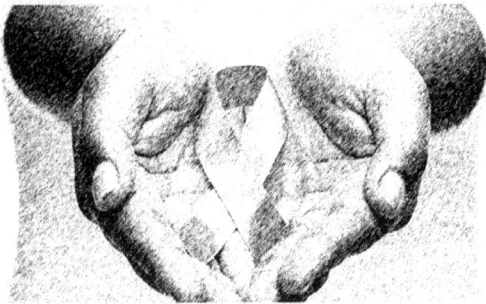

It has been a while since I have practiced medicine. Sometimes I feel as if I had abandoned the battlefield, leaving my mission unfinished, but I know it is due to the emptiness that invades us when we stop playing such a demanding and important role. For this reason, I decided to write this book and share my experience. It is also my intention to share some thoughts about the human being, and the circumstances around us when we are "behind the scenes of cancer", with our needs, victories and frustrations. If this book can be of help to a single person, whether a physician, or a patient, or their families, I will have accomplished another step in my mission on Earth and this will comfort me deeply.

When I chose to be a doctor and specializing in oncology, I wanted to help people and to improve my understanding of human nature. I always studied and worked with this target in mind, more than anything else. I had the illusion that better knowing the functioning of the body would make my life more fulfilling and useful. In my home country, where a significant portion of the population lives in poverty, the dream of helping people out is quite common, devoid of any heroic connotation. The low quality of life and the harsh conditions are troubling, and encourage us to take action; but the poor were not my only subjects, of course.

Today, I no longer live in a country where poverty rules, but I still feel the call to help people — poor people in a wider sense, because we all share the poverty of human limitations.

It is not my intention to be didactic, because I am not a teacher. All I want is to express my thoughts in a straightforward language, even colloquial, and I hope my work will generate a constructive interaction among readers and the people around them.

With my patients, I learned many lessons. I also suffered through the experience of having a family member affected by cancer, and in this battle, I lost my beloved sister. Unfortunately, in her case, breast cancer was not detected at an early stage, despite all the information available to such an intelligent and educated person, despite the presence of an oncologist by her side, to whom she could have asked for help. When she finally did, the cancer had already spread to the regional lymph nodes and the prognosis was not so good. Nevertheless, even if the conditions were far from ideal, the treatment allowed her another 10 years of living well, without signs of the disease. The chance of metastasis existed, though; and unfortunately, they happened.

I am telling you all these facts to emphasize the importance of early diagnosis. If we can detect cancer in the very beginning of its development, the possibility of cure is higher. It is therefore essential to pass screening tests periodically. Self-examination is also very useful in the case of breast cancer. All women should be examined regularly.

I invite you to ask your doctor in order to get informed about the procedures available and recommended for you, as a prevention or in the eventuality of a treatment. Each case of cancer must be evaluated carefully, because there are many distinct situations. Cancer may develop completely different behaviors, depending on multiple circumstances. We cannot generalize.

During my years as a doctor, I worked with the rich and the poor, the young and the old, the educated and the less educated. I am quite sure I have a rich testimony to offer, I am very conscious of that. I dare say I have accumulated so many hours next to the suffering, deeply involved in the fight for life, that I am ready to venture into some considerations about it. But I do not wish to tell tearful stories. Reality is hard enough; we do not need to add further pain.

I know cancer patients like to learn about their disease. They frequently ask many questions, and I think I can help, giving them a general idea of some basic concepts. I am also convinced that sharing our feelings and experiences is an effective way to help each other and to make the suffering less heavy to bear. Having fought this disease on both sides (professionally and in my family), I want to continue to contribute as much as I can and in any way I am allowed to (I have not managed to get a medical license in Quebec, more about that later).

As the French saying goes: "*En méde-*

*cine comme en amour, ni jamais ni toujours*"[1] — I do not know the author, but how true it is! A teacher from my Medical College uttered this citation as a first lesson we should never forget. I still remember; and whatever I say in this book is not definitive. We do not know the laws that govern the universe; we are very far from knowing them all. We are in a continuous learning process and it is in this condition that I share my thoughts. I do not admit it out of humbleness; but because that's how I see our reality: We are always learning.

The topics are all open to discussion. Sometimes I ask questions that border philosophy... a mental exercise everyone should do. Therefore, I invite you to think critically about each issue on which I focus, and you will see that the benefit of reading this book will be much larger; you will be creating something new with your own talents and, perhaps, new ideas will emerge.

Knowledge, science, or ideas — it doesn't matter how we call our experience — everything evolves from the learning acquired previously, which opens a door to a new room; in this manner, we will explore unknown labyrinths.

---

1 In Medicine as in love, never say never, never say always.

## 2. Cancer - A New Approach

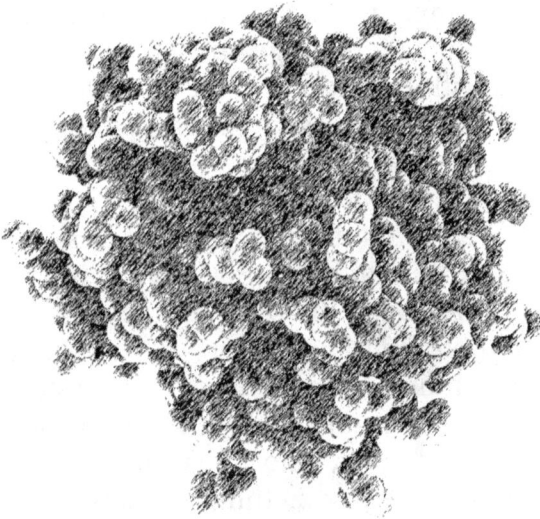

What is the origin of the word cancer? This designation is credited to the Greek physician Hippocrates (460-370 BC), who is considered the "father of medicine". Hippocrates used the terms *carcinos* and *carcinoma* to describe tumors. In Greek these words refer to the crab, and are related to the visual appearance of the disease, because the finger-like projections formed during the propagation from the initial lesion resemble the shape of a crab. The Roman physician Aulus Cornelius Celsus (25 BC-50 AD) translated the Greek word to "cancer", the Latin word for crab. Galen (130-200 AD), another Roman physician of Greek origin, used the word *oncos* (swelling, in Greek) to describe these tumors. While the analogy of Hippocrates and Celsus with the crab is still used to describe malignant tumors, the term of Galen is now often used as a reference to cancer specialists — the oncologists.

With an introduction like this, this text does seem didactic. But, no, this is not a medical textbook. It is rather a personal reflection on the topic, as I try to get a better understanding of humans and the circumstances surrounding us, in order to move forward. However, before sharing my ideas, I need to explain something about the basic mechanism by which cancer develops and spreads, based on what we know about this disease.

I will try to use a simple language. Even if the text, sometimes, seems to have too many technicalities, that could only be of interest for people specialized in the area, please, try to read it patiently, because all I write in this book can be useful for everybody, and it helps knowing more about this increasingly widespread disease.

First of all, it is important to talk briefly about our body tissues, because there's a similarity between cancer cells and embryonic cells, concerning their character of growth. Yes, it is true! So, let's move on... When the ovum from the mother and the spermatozoon from the father join to give birth to the human egg, they form a totipotent cell. Totipotent means "with all potential"; totipotent because this cell has everything it needs to develop all body tissues; in other words, from this cell a human being will be formed, with different tissues — for example, the skin tissue will be distinct from the liver tissue, and different from the brain tissue... and so on and so forth. But all these different cells in the human body were initially a unique cell, with all the features not yet differentiated into distinct tissues.

As a parenthesis, I should add a note on semantics. You must have noticed a word that might be unknown to many of you, "totipotent". Yes, this word exists, and is present in major dictionaries! It is widely used when discussing embryology, and also oncology. I think it is irreplaceable, and that is why I have not tried any synonyms. Furthermore, I like this term, because when we refer to the "totipotency," we transmit the magnitude of the idea. "Toti" comes from the Latin "*totus*" and means entire, complete. "Potent" also from Latin, means powerful. The meaning of "totipotent" is impressive: The totipotent cell has "everything it takes," it has the power to form a complete being.

Gradually, as the cells multiply in the embryonic phase, the newest ones are subject to influences that make them differentiate. Thus, they begin to agglomerate here and there; as they accumulate, they take the form of organs and tissue masses. In general, when they become differentiated, they lose the ability to be totipotent, i.e., they become increasingly specialized in certain functions. For example, liver tissue produces substances the skin does not… And so it goes.

All normal cells have a system in charge of the cell division process, a combination of stimulation and inhibition of the cell multiplication, conducted by genes (proto-oncogene/ oncogene, anti-oncogene etc.) — to simplify the text I will call it the "O complex."

Now, let us talk about cancer… For some reason (sometimes known, sometimes not), a cell (or a few cells) of a body tissue undergoes a change, for example, a mutation, which triggers the process of cell division without the usual controls. Often, the cellular machinery is able to fix the problem, but in other cases, it is not, and this is how the cancer cell appears. The cancer cell begins to multiply without the normal "O complex" control, which becomes faulty. The cancer cell multiplies without complying with the laws that govern its healthy environment. The cell seems to return to a more ancient stage, i.e., it mutates into a cell with more undifferentiated characteristics. It apparently goes back to a younger stage, similar to the embryonic phase, where it used to multiply itself more actively. Sometimes it loses much of its differentiation, of its specialization. However, it still retains some of its characteristics, because the behavior of the disease varies, depending on the tissue where the cancer originates.

It is important to mention that cancer is not a uniform disease; it manifests itself in several forms. The multiplication rate often depends on the degree of cell differentiation. This cell reproduction, apparently without control, forms masses of cells that increase in volume and turn into tumors, clusters of cells that no longer behave as normal tissue, with cells working together, in concert with the rest of the organism. They do not even respect their territory, and have a tendency to be independent and to invade adjacent tissues; they tend to lose the cohesion with the original tissue, acquiring the propensity to move away and go elsewhere, settling far from their original place (their location said "primitive") where they continue to multiply (metastasis).

In short, chaos takes charge. This whole process consumes a lot of nutrients, and the energy of the affected person, with no apparent purpose. The masses of cells grow faster than the body is able to feed them, and many of them perish during the growing process, releasing toxic substances. These tumors can also produce undesirable mechanical effects, such as compressions and obstructions. All these events may lead to the patient's death, if we do nothing to retake control of the situation.

Countless studies and theories try to explain this bizarre behavior of the cancer cell, and the reasons why the body fails to control it. Several genetic alterations (hereditary and nonhereditary) were detected in this process; but the primary cause, why it happens, it is not yet known. Why does the "O complex" of a cell change, in order to allow this limitless multiplication? We look for reasons here and there, but the mystery is still greater than the findings. We also know that there are many factors helping the appearance of the disease, such as: certain habits; certain foods, or how we eat them; the exposure to toxic agents; and the combination of these and many other factors. But the real reason remains unknown.

When we finally manage to discover what's behind the cancer mechanism, then we will find an effective cure for the disease. Definitely, the elimination of some factors does help tremendously. For example, it is a proven fact that the habit of smoking is an important risk factor for developing lung cancer. It does not act alone, of course; the person at risk has other factors working together. Yet, probably, to many of these people, not smoking is the factor protecting them against lung cancer; but avoiding risk factors is not nearly enough.

I will exemplify with an analogy: suppose there is a hidden hole on one side of a field, and plenty of fruits a wild animal likes to eat all around it. If the animal goes to that side of the field to eat those fruits, it has a greater probability of falling down into that hole. There is also a chance it does not fall. If we remove the fruits, the chance of the animal going there is reduced, but it can go anyway; and still fall down. In order to completely prevent the risk of falling down the hole, we must eliminate the hole itself! Since the hole is actually hidden from everyone, preventive measures and the treatment of cancer are all peripheral, i.e., they never reach the center of the enigma.

What is the strategy of existing treatments, such as chemotherapy? They are conceived to attack the cells in their process of cellular division. The drug molecules either behave as fraudulent components of the cell structure, or they poison inner cell elements needed for the process of multiplication, just to mention an example. Consequently, cancer cells are killed in the act of division. As we know, cancer cells multiply quickly; and this strategy affects them in large numbers.

In my opinion, there is a serious problem with this kind of logistics. Even if it is considered a very advanced and clever method, aiming the cell division in its intimate path, like we do in most existing treatments, has the unique goal of killing cancer cells that are multiplying quickly. In addition, the treatment also kills other cells of the body that have a normal high rate of multiplication, and this is the cause of most of the side effects. For example, the bone marrow cells, responsible for the fabrication of blood cells, are affected directly, because they multiply quickly. The consequence is a smaller production of blood cells. This can lead to anemia (low red blood cells count), hemorrhages (due to low platelet count) and to infections (due to leucopenia, a low count of white blood cells, the "soldiers" of the body, that protect us against infectious agents; with a low count of these soldiers, the body become more susceptible to infections).

These consequences can be dangerous, configuring most serious conditions, frequently life threatening and demanding prompt intervention.

Another example of quickly multiplying cells is the hair matrix epithelium, one of the fastest growing cell populations in the human body; this is the reason why the treatment may lead to temporary hair loss.

Currently, there are some tricks to target cancer cells exclusively, but these tricks are not available in all drugs and yet, they do not affect the primary cause. One "crazy" cell may remain untouched, able to resume its pace, or it can develop equal "tricks" to continue its propagation, which is called "resistance mechanism."

Therefore, we continue to see adverse side effects, despite the entire arsenal trying to circumvent them. And yet we continue to see recurrences of the disease, on short or long term. Without forgetting cancer that is secondary to treatment, which develops from the carcinogenic action of the treatment itself.

We know there are new studies leading to the creation of drugs with innovative mechanisms: in a simple and clear language, one of them has the purpose of making cancer cells "visible" for our immune system (again the strategy is to make war between cells); another one is supposed to target the mutation which triggers the acceleration of cell division. Neither of those seems to me to be "Egg of Columbus."

I believe no drug has yet reached the primary cause of cancer because cancer cells have the ability to thwart treatment by their resistance mechanisms. They undergo changes to continue their inexorable journey, their vicious tendency to multiply. What is the origin of this trend?

Meanwhile, the patients are there, they must be treated as quickly as possible, with the tools we have in hand. Still, this treatment manages to achieve surprising results; more and more cases are in long-term remission, we can even say, "cured."

Nevertheless, in terms of research, in addition to working with the new drugs designed to kill cells, we could perhaps think of **a new approach**. I know it is hard to think out of the box, because our universe, this visible universe, leads us to death, and the weapons we are able to create are designed to kill, in accordance with the laws of nature — "kill to survive," is the available motto in all levels.

If this statement scares you, and if you refuse to accept our predatory reality, you are, like me, taking the first steps towards the vision of another dimension; but that is another story...

### A new approach

With all the progress in the study of genes in recent years, there must be a way to scrutinize these cells more effectively, subjecting them to environments similar to the human body, in order to interact with the mechanisms of cell division. This would change the notion of testing substances to destroy the dividing cell, or circumventing the situation with "tricks," because the cell also responds with "tricks". We cannot forget we are in a system where the principle that prevails is that of action and reaction (to every action there is always opposed an equal reaction). And if we started to play with the cell's ability to multiply? We should try to put this cell back in its "good behavior," returning to its normal pace and respecting the laws that govern its environment — this is the "new approach" I'm talking about.

If we develop such studies, perhaps we will find many more responses than expected. Maybe, by studying the origin of the cancer cell behavior, we could learn more about our very nature, about the laws that govern us, the standard behavior within our reach for now — life → growth → death — under the command of this perpetual motion of actions and reactions.

In the previous paragraphs, I explained

the behavior of embryonic cells and of cancer cells in order to highlight the similarities in their character of growth. In principle, this is not an intrinsic behavior of "death." Somehow, this process reproduces, in accelerated mode, the pattern of nature: We come to life, we grow up, and then we die. We need to thwart this standard, this vicious circle. I invite you all to think about this striking reality.

### Brainstorming

Now, another parenthesis is required... This book has already borne a small fruit, as I interacted with my family. That is exactly what I want: We shall think together and launch our ideas. I add here a small step forward; maybe it will encourage others.

Talking with my brother Francisco, an engineer, about the cancer cell, he gave a sequence to my thoughts in a different and surprising way! I think it is perfectly logical. When I shared my thoughts with him, he reasoned the following: "The mutation which triggers the cancer cell behavior of growth could be a vital reaction to repair a damage."

Suddenly, the sequence of cancer development started to make sense! Let us follow attentively the possible concatenation of events: A potentially lethal agent — a carcinogen, like radiation, for example — attacks a normal cell, that is damaged to such an extent that it mutates. This mutation, apparently random, may have the purpose of repairing the destructive effect experienced by the cell, i.e., this change triggers the mechanism of cell division. In this way, the "desperate" multiplication of the cells could target the replacement of damaged cells, considered by the system as dying cells. It would be a pro-life reaction!

### The Proposition

What in this book we call the "O complex" is the genetic component (or the genetic components) responsible for conducting the process of cell division — we must keep an eye on it! If we identify this kind of reaction, and if we manage to control it, we will be able to stop a case of cancer! And, in other cases, this phenomenon could be useful, as, for instance, a source of tissue renewal; maybe a way of renewing life itself!

What we have proposed at this moment is an idea: To develop a treatment that can control the tumor progression without using tricks to kill the cells; i.e., a process that does not perpetuate reactions to aggressive actions. To achieve this goal, it is necessary to study the "O Complex" more closely, in order to try to control it or, perhaps, strengthen it somehow; and thus reversing the process of "despair" in cell multiplication.

Life force is very intense, and in the case of cancer, not properly adjusted. We will not be able to repair this wrong adjustment trying to eliminate it with all the violence and naiveté of current treatments. We must find another way.

I know we are far from being able to play with this phenomenon. However, we should at least think about this possibility. The task at hand will be enormous, I know, but we need to rethink it again and again. With small steps — because our legs are short — we will succeed in this journey, despite its length; and when we reach the end of the way, we will pass the baton to someone else, as in a relay race.

I passed my baton by writing this book. Now it is your turn…

## 3. THE PATIENT

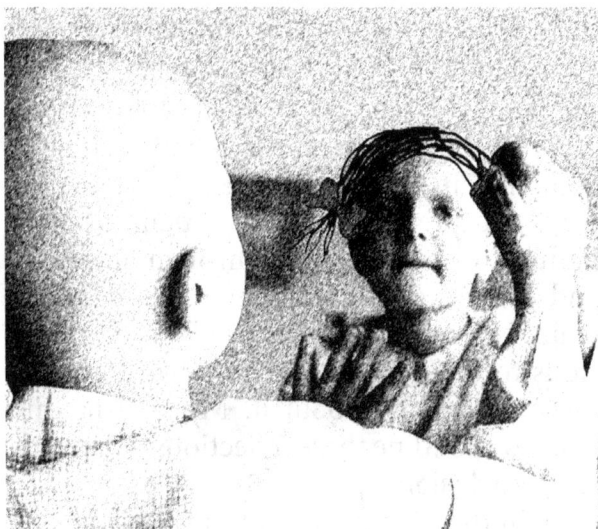

*102 Reasons*

*I write for you*
*The true words.*
*Your shiny eyes*
 *I wanted to paint*
*Most beautiful eyes.*
*If the gray clouds frighten you*

*Look at my flowers*
*Today they are hope*
*The garden is full of promise.*
*I'm here*
*By your side*
*I'm singing a hundred notes*
*And two more.*
*I count and recount*
*The reasons to keep my 102 flowers garden.*
*I plant them for you.*

During my years of practice, I have compiled in my memory several types of feelings expressed, either by patients or their families, or by caregivers, through questions and comments, compliments and complaints... Finally, I gathered all the impressions received in this environment to create my own feelings about it. My goal in this work is to outline these reflections; I dare not say "conclusions."

In this chapter, I want to tell you about those to whom I have dedicated much of my life — my oncology patients; and for them I would like to deliver a message of hope. I still think about helping them, as I give them my support throughout this text. I also invite their families and friends, and also physicians and all the health care team to read it, because it can be interesting and useful for all.

I take inspiration from these people who are the more important element in the "trio" disease/ doctor/ patient. Doctors exist to take care of the patients; and the disease exists as well because the patients are there, with all the special and unique circumstances involving each one.

The word 'patient', as used in Medicine, concerns the person who receives the action, being the passive element. That's exactly how we often see those people arriving at the office with a recent cancer diagnosis — in shock, unable to properly manage their own ideas. They suddenly feel completely devoid of power, incapable of deciding about their own life; an unexpected illness has taken control. In addition, tests are needed, there is an endless list of exams... and they are urgent! Treatment must start as quickly as possible!

With all the access to information, made easier for everybody through the internet, it is not a secret that cancer is curable in many cases. The adverse side effects of the treatment are increasingly controllable; nevertheless, the fear of cancer is still strong and present. Death suddenly appears in the mirror, a terrible event; even if it is the only certainty we have on Earth. Some people affirm that death does not scare them, but they do not want to face the pain and suffering.

I think this is in fact a tardive reaction, in a more accepting phase, when reasoning comes into play. I believe the initial shock, following the diagnosis, is caused by the confrontation with the possibility of dying, which incites the survival instinct.

Survival instinct usually leads us to perform a sequence of reflex actions, in order to keep us alive; but when it comes to a serious disease like cancer, patients are forced to delegate this privilege to someone else, and the doctor becomes their main "survival tool." Individual reactions vary, but in most cases, that's how it happens. At this moment, without realizing it, patients establish an instinctive link with their savior — or saviors, since the treatment is often multidisciplinary, i.e., there are several disciplines involved: surgery, chemotherapy and radiation therapy, among others. And each discipline has its own specialist.

Now, we have an important point to consider. In this diversified, new universe for most people, patients can feel as if they were in a labyrinth, an additional factor for the sensation of being lost, even after the consultation with the doctor. It's too much to digest in such a short period of time. I think it is very important to have someone in the multidisciplinary team who will talk more frequently with the patients, to explain all the details, to answer their questions throughout the treatment.

Sometimes, it is possible for the oncologist to play this important role; but doctors are usually too busy in making decisions, choosing between highly technical choices, in order to obtain the best results, and they are rarely able to perform this extra task. Some may be capable of doing it, in less busy departments of oncology, but I think it is not the rule, and the presence of someone else to fulfill this important supporting role is mandatory. If patients have very specific questions related to the treatment, that person may act as an intermediary between patients and their doctor, if an immediate appointment is not possible. It is desirable to take note of all coordinates in this meeting, since they may very well be necessary.

In most modern oncology centers, these specific attendants are often nurses or social workers. Sometimes, psychologists are required, but only in more specific, unusual cases. In the hospital where I worked, after several years of experience, our team adopted the multidisciplinary model, in which oncologists are responsible for the patients, of course, but in concert with other professionals that have the same importance.

I mention this multidisciplinary model because I've got good results in this kind of practice; but, certainly, there are other similar valid experiences. The key to the success, in my opinion, is the constant support for the patient, because it is a very demanding treatment, sometimes with considerable complications. In addition, patients and their families should be informed about everything, in order to face the battle with the disposition and preparation needed, not as a passive element. Thus, we manage to avoid surprises that might destabilize the entire structure.

In some cases, however, patients do not want to receive information; they develop an almost impenetrable barrier, almost palpable — it is not difficult to detect this trick, and I believe we must respect this reaction. If we try to demolish the patient's defense, the results can be disastrous. Psychologists would be more appropriate to better explain this phenomenon, and take charge of such cases. I saw it happen quite often during my years of practice; I observed oncologists as they smashed the locked door, and the result was not pleasant. I do not dare to force a door closed by someone in a state of suffering; we must give this person time.

On the other hand, for someone who wants to learn more about the disease and its treatment, in addition to the instructions provided directly by the health care team, there are plenty of reliable websites widely available. It is necessary, though, to find a reliable source of information. I recommend the Canadian Cancer Society website.[2]

I also invite you to read the section entitled "The Call," at the end of this chapter.

### *The role of the family and friends*

When talking about patients, we cannot forget their families and friends, because the role of people around them is very important. When in need, we take great comfort in our loved ones. It is easier to face difficulties when we have the help of people around us. The disease and its treatment become a weight less heavy to bear. For the patient, it is also a way to experience the humility of being part of this universe, part of its development, allowing others to mature through their good deeds. How comforting it is for the family and friends to be an auxiliary instrument! How rewarding it is to be present, to say kind words, to help as much as possible, and then think of yourself as someone who has accomplished a mission! And not for the sake of obligation, but just out love, yes, it is infinitely comforting.

For those who do not feel concerned when someone close to them becomes ill,

2 http://www.cancer.ca/

think about it: all of us will have our own time of need, when the help of others will be welcomed. Keeping ourselves unscathed throughout life is a very rare event; it is simply a matter of time. And if we do not help our loved ones, perhaps we are at risk of not receiving help when we need it. I don't say that as a threat, it is only logical: if we are not present for someone in need, there's a chance this person will forget us as well — that's reality, that's how it works. Even if we are very rich, and have many people to take care of us, it is not the same as being surrounded by true friends and family.

It is worthy of emphasis that, in helping each other, we are acting together to develop a better world, for everybody. Every action leads to a reaction, and in this case it is not different.

### *Write away your feelings*

The information given by the health care team is not the only one that matters. Some notes taken by the patients can be very useful at times, to the doctors and to other caregivers. Patients can write a kind of journal, with all the comments they deem important, regarding their symptoms and changes observed during the treatment. It will be certainly of good use for everyone. At the same time, they can make a list of questions they want to ask to their oncology team on their coming appointment.

When many questions and conflicts arise, we tend to forget some of them. The checklist will help to reduce this common anxiety. Additionally, patients can write their personal impressions, deliver a testimony to share their experience with others, as I'm doing now. Sharing is always welcome.

### *Feeling guilty?*

When the patient is a child, or a teenager, there is an extra reason to justify the need for psychological support, not only for them, but also for their families. Young patients are not necessarily aware of their own death, but several issues will arise during treatment, such as the alterations in their self-image and the special care and attention they will need as well; in other words, they will face major changes in their lives. For the family, especially for the parents, this support is essential, because they often feel more affected by their children's pain than by their own. In addition to their own suffering as parents, they also absorb that of their children.

Sometimes the effect on parents is so

catastrophic that their despair is noticeable by the children, and transmitted to them. We should avoid such trouble at all costs, because it can disrupt the relationship with caregivers and, consequently, disturb the progress of the treatment. Young patients often become irritable and intolerant; it seems that they feel guilty for being the cause of their parents' suffering, and they just want to stop it. This way, the scenario becomes even more painful.

Parents do not need to prove their love of their children, showing off their despair because of the child's illness. Greater proof of love is to support them with serenity, to make them feel good.

Sometimes, another issue occurs. Parents transfer a vague feeling of guilt to the health care team, and it's not easy to deal with this. Parents may feel as if they made some mistake in their child's life, and they are unable to accept they did something wrong. Guilt is too heavy for them to bear, and they instinctively transfer it to the health care team. Usually, there is no such thing as wrongdoing; it is rather a matter of discomfort caused by the disease. We must pay attention to this kind of problem.

Childhood is a singular phenomenon in itself. I have so many questions about it that go beyond the medical field. Simplistic physiologic answers are not enough for me; there is something unexplainable in this state of development, something we must respect with all due astonishment. But as this topic is not the target of this book, I leave it for later.

### *Immortality*

In my opinion, when adults are ill, regardless of their social class or level of education, they react in a similar pattern — paradoxically, each one in their unique way, because each person is unique, but everyone has a point in common, and nothing for now can change it: the unavoidable death. Although wealth and education can provide a little more comfort and understanding of the situation, they make no difference when it comes to confronting death, this event that befalls to us all, without distinction.

Usually, we do not think we are going to die, although it is the only certainty we have in life — this solitary finitude —, in its universality. Each one fights for survival in their own way, as if it were a quest for immortality, an idea that haunts us and confronts us continuously.

This search for the cure of diseases, these efforts to obtain an increased life expectancy… is it a human tendency to just go further, in order to reach immortality? Why not? Why do life and death exist? Where is the origin of life's vicious circle? And why do we keep this ancestral survival instinct?

### Coming back to Earth

Let us come back, down to Earth... It is important to consider each person's disposition. The ideal is to keep patients functional during and after treatment. If they have a good supply of health, if the disease and the treatment do not prevent them from keeping up with their daily activities, I think they should continue their life as normally as possible. But the doctor is not alone in making these decisions; patients will also establish their own limits.

However, during the cancer treatment, the patient's immune system often becomes compromised. The host defense to infectious agents weakens, and the patient is prone to an increased risk of acquiring infections. In these cases, in order to avoid exposition to this risk, isolation could be necessary, mainly during critical periods. The doctor will determine assessments to help the patients to protect themselves.

Even if isolated, risks may continue to threaten the patient, since microorganisms present in the body can take advantage of the situation, i.e., the weakened defenses can allow opportunistic agents to start acting. It is very important to follow the guidelines of the health care team; but paranoia is not recommended. Today, medicine has the means to counter the consequences of an intensely decreased host defense, and there are drugs designed to stimulate the production of defense cells. Oncologists have now a large arsenal of measures and drugs to counter the side effects of the treatment, which has become much less painful than in the past. The need for hospital admission, for example, dropped substantially.

By the way, hair loss is one of the most feared side effects, and there is not much to do in order to avoid it. Self-image is a very important point to consider, it is undeniable. The face and the hair are the first trace of a person's identity. Hair loss is thus an additional loss, added to the difficult conditions already experienced by the patients. This is not trivial, as one could argue. Losing hair so abruptly is a real aggression, and if the patient's well-being is at stake, it is necessary to address this situation. We must consider all the chances for success; I think a wig is quite a satisfactory solution, and it can be commissioned, in order to reproduce the normal look of the person as accurately as possible.

The intention is not to hide the truth, but to eliminate unnecessary suffering. Every effort must be made to keep the patient's spirit high, this is crucial in order to guarantee good results. *Voilà!*

With the progress of treatment, an increasingly growing number of cases are becoming curable. We must get rid of the preconceived idea that equates cancer to death; this is not always the case. And positive thinking always adds motivation for a battle that will lead to victory.

Sometimes, we find ourselves alone with our thoughts and doubts. We must not isolate ourselves from others; the ideal is to seek help, to reach out for more information, to talk with someone. It is important not to get discouraged. I know it is not easy; it is one of the reasons for writing this book. I want to be there for you, as an auxiliary tool to assist those seeking motivation not to give up, those in search for answers, trying to understand what is happening to them... I also try my best to understand the circumstances surrounding us; and I chose to write in this informal style, that allows us to open our "thinking box."

I do not offer miraculous solutions; all I want is to share my thoughts with you, and to be at your side at this time of probation.

However, if you think this is not the

time for questioning, for a deep reflection, if you feel like changing the subject, listen to your heart; leave this reading for another time. Perhaps, it is necessary to engage yourself in an activity that gives you pleasure, something that makes you feel better. We all need a break to "recharge our batteries."

What is important is to keep the morals up, to help us face the situation.

### And here we go...

As for the treatment itself, even in the most complicated and difficult situations, I would never say we have lost the battle. All of a sudden, science may find how to proceed to ease the trap in which the body falls, as it allows the development of cancer — I firmly believe in that. And I mean the real trap, not factors that increase or diminish possibilities, making the field more or less favorable to the disease.

One day, we still do not know how or when, we will find the key to open the door to a complete cure. And if this happens tomorrow? With this idea in mind, I was always motivated to persist, to go on treating even the more resistant cases, those with less favorable prognosis. Once the treatment was fighting the disease, being no more threatening to the patient than the disease itself, I never wanted to stop; and I explained this mindset to the patients and their families. I was always ready to continue, and it was up to them to decide differently.

This remains clear in my mind: each patient should be considered the main element motivating doctors as they decide in favor of a treatment. It does not matter how much the health care system need to invest; all effort must be done in order to obtain the best results. Even if it seems too obvious, I insist, I emphasize it. We are the reflection of each other, "in image and likeness." When we take care of a person and observe the results, it is always a learning process, an accomplishment for all. It is one more step to know better the universe that exists inside each one of us, representing the totality. This is how I see things.

Yes, patients are the most important parameter in this equation; all other elements must adjust to their needs. Then, with the experience we acquired, we will adapt the treatment to each individual, and this will be part of a new estimation, which will establish the basis of future treatment guidelines. Our actions and decisions will be useful for ourselves, and for everybody else.

The decision as to when we should halt cancer treatment in less favorable cases is not unanimous, even among patients. In my opinion, this should be a joint decision involving doctors and patients — or their representative —, after open discussion with both sides.

### Beliefs

Despite the need for all this meticulous care, maybe because of it, oncology patients find themselves in the midst of a real battle, it is undeniable; and sometimes they are tempted to seek alternative treatments. More often than not, patients and their families will hear about some treatment considered "not orthodox" by conventional medicine, such as "miraculous" drugs or methods, surprisingly not yet known by science, and promising a high cure rate.

I have seen a few, who previously counted themselves among the more skeptical, engage in this kind of thing when a family member is affected by cancer, or in case they are a cancer patient themselves. Even I, when my sister was considered incurable, found myself tempted to believe in such treatments, suggested by people around me. I figured, if the considered substance wasn't likely to cause any harm to the organism, and if it could not jeopardize the official treatment, there would be no problem in taking it. Basically, there was the germ of hoping this "treatment" could have a beneficial effect, and I don't say it because I experienced it. The phenomenon is neither new nor rare; it is a common reaction that should not be envisioned as a serious mistake, especially when we know that many treatments existing today originated from trivial observations, not always in highly equipped laboratories.

As a physician, when I was still steeped in the omnipotence of doctors as holders of the power to diagnose and cure, before my family was touched by cancer, I used to find this quest for supposedly miraculous treatments ridiculous. I have been many times intolerant toward this kind of attitude coming from patients and their families, and I admit it. "*Errare humanum est*," says the famous Latin citation.

We must at all costs avoid going to extremes; neither should we abandon the treatment prescribed by the doctor to venture in the taking of unknown and poorly studied substances, nor should we completely deny them, *a priori*. The judgement must always be based on the priorities. If it is for the sake of mind calming that hope brings, the use of these substances is to be considered on the menu; at the same time, we need to explain clearly, to the patients and their families, the real reason for its use.

We do need to believe in something. It seems that this tendency to have beliefs is innate to the human being — a religion or an ideal can feed our needs in that direction. How small we become, when we choose to ignore the power of faith! We do not have enough knowledge to judge anything in this domain. Besides, we know science itself is still largely based upon beliefs. Even if it is always trying to present evidence, we know very well how concepts, once clearly demonstrated and considered untouchable, may suffer from a sudden fall, when faced with new findings — it has happened many times in the history of science.

Why do we have this serious deviation, to believe that we know the truth? All we have is a few beliefs... always! Even the skeptics, who believe in nothing, believe in themselves. And again, it is only another belief...

### In the waiting room

When speaking about my main character's environment, I still have something to add: life is not always rosy in the waiting rooms of the oncology departments, it is easy to figure that out. Please, do not forget we are all similar, but we have our own particularities, we should never generalize.

Cancer can show itself in many different ways, depending on the cell from which it originates, according to the phase (in oncology, we often say "stage"), and especially depending on the host. Finally, we could say there are several different diseases called "cancer." The scenarios we come upon in an oncology department include a wide variety of situations. The health status and the appearance of a given person is not a step that all affected will forcefully face, we cannot project ourselves perfectly onto another's image, since the contours do not fit. The predictable is not always visible.

Therefore, do not feed your imagination with bad scenarios. We are unique, and we have our own personal way of reacting to the injury and its treatment.

### The Call

As I said previously, I would like to invite everyone to participate in creating a new project, the new approach to cancer I mentioned in Chapter 2. Patients are always the priority, and they should not keep a passive attitude. As the carriers of a lesion — that might eventually become the light at the end of the tunnel —, patients' contribution is essential in the search for a way-out, a solution for all humankind. According to the project's progress at the time of their contribution, patients could already benefit from the results themselves.

Obviously, I am not suggesting that anyone neglects the treatment currently underway, to venture as a Paladin in search of fantastic solutions. The proposition is to act according to each one's availability, as simple as that. For those whose only contact with a vehicle of science is the doctor, and the health care team, goes my advice to share with them our ideas, in case they have not engaged yet; even better for those with access to college research centers or pharmaceutical companies.

The starting point is to propose studies that will be able to generate treatments whose mechanisms of action will not include the death of the cell among its main objectives — this is, in my opinion, the "magic recipe." This idea is outlined in the sections "A new approach" and "The Proposition," both in Chapter 2.

There will be some resistance from scientists, certainly; but we can't give up easily. Ask your doctors to, at least, launch this idea in the next medical conference they attend, as a message from a patient — there may be someone who cares. If necessary, we can offer for research some tissue samples, normal or pathological. The broader the sampling is, the greater the reliability of the study will be.

We are in the era of social networks, and they are quite effective in disseminating so many events, so many stories... We can use them for this purpose as well. I will also use social networks to propagate my ideas.

We need to accelerate the studies on cancer, to extend their range of possibilities, so that treatments become less aggressive and more effective. It takes further effort to innovate, much more research than has already been done is necessary. Many advances have been accomplished, but they are still far from enough. Hundreds of years had passed us by, and the complete cure for cancer has not been achieved...

Let us act upon it. We all share the same boat. Let's set sail, then!

# 4. The Medical Doctor

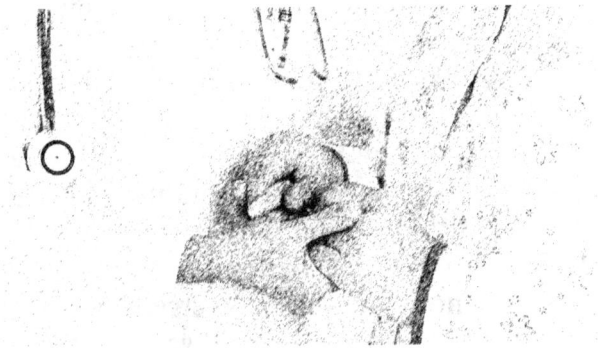

The medical doctor: who is this guy? Who is this person, who desires to be a healer?

The dictionary tells us it is someone trained in the healing arts and licensed to practice them. Since the dawn of time, all human communities, even the most primitive, had counted on someone to treat sick people, sometimes considered a kind of magician or sorcerer, with supernatural powers.

The concepts have changed, but there is still today a reminder of this old belief; we still consider doctors must have a "vocation," a "calling," a special talent, in order to practice their profession. At least, doctors must be performing students, since in most countries the access to Medical School is reserved for those with better grades, or the ones who succeed in the difficult exams to enter college. It is understandable, because doctors will take care of the most important asset we have, the very thing that will keep us alive — our health.

We take for granted the concept that the search for healing is a logical idea; but if we give it some thought, if we try to free our mind from its previous conditioning, we will see in this attitude a special attempt to thwart the perishable nature of our universe, what we know about the universe.

In fact, doctors are always working against the current; their purpose is to reverse the natural processes that make us perish. In this sense, until today it is expected from doctors a vocation to the supernatural, not far from the sorcerer of primitive tribes. I say "supernatural" in its strictest meaning, of course, that is to say, beyond the laws of nature (of this universe, as we know it).

Of course, in order to treat sick people, the doctors have at their disposal only tools created in this same universe, and subject to the same laws. It does not change the fact it is an action to counter our perishable nature —

it seems paradoxical, and I say, "seems," because we know so little about ourselves that it would be arrogant to cultivate certainties.

One question keeps coming to my mind, and I am relieved to share it with you, because it is also a call for reflection, a search for answers I am not yet able to find. Maybe while reading this book someone will go one step further, in the quest for solutions. This question is about the conflict I observe between the concept that we belong in this perishable world and our propensity to escape it. The search for healing, the efforts to increase life expectancy, would that be a sign, perhaps, that finitude does not serve us? That our integrity does not belong in this pattern offered by this perishable universe, as we know it?

Back to our magicians/ sorcerers who are trying to heal: As there is so much technology available to help them today, I would say they are now professionals of the industry, but, fortunately, medical intuition never loses its place.

Why does one choose the medical profession? What motivates a young student to decide to go into this area? I can answer this question in part. When I chose to be a doctor, I wanted to know the human being more deeply and try to help people. My father was a doctor, and I cannot say he did not influence me. He was a highly skilled and dedicated physician, and he practiced charitably; he was considered a blessed person.

In a country where there was (and there still is) a large portion of the population living in poverty, as is the case of my home country, and at a time when the health care system was not as bureaucratized as today, he has dedicated his life to helping others. For sure, people like him strongly influence those around them, but I never thought my choice was because of him, because I never dreamed to be like him — this idea never irrupted in my consciousness. As strange as it may seem, it is now, as I write this work, that this idea occurs to me for the first time.

Why does one choose to be an oncologist? People often asked me this question.

First, what is an oncologist? The oncologist is a physician who treats patients diagnosed with cancer. The current trend is to form specialists in each field, i.e., surgical oncology, radiotherapy, clinical or medical oncology, and pediatric oncology — the latter two involving treatment with drugs. All of them are part of a larger oncology team.

In my case, I did an internship in a department of clinical oncology, and I liked it. I found it very well organized, and I ended up doing my specialization in the same department. Then I was invited to stay in the team, and now I take this opportunity to pay tribute to our tutor in the oncology department, Dr. Sebastião Cabral Filho, M.D. Dr. Cabral is also the head of the Center to Antiblastic Chemotherapy and Immunotherapy, where I worked for twenty years.[3] He is a very competent and dynamic person, always interested in spreading knowledge and the pleasure of studying.

I remember when we complained about not having enough time to study, because we took care of sick people all day and had only the evening to study. Here is his advice: "What do you do at night? Go study!" And he was right. We must study a lot, we must give our hearts and souls! When I was young, it was said Medicine was like a priesthood, and it sure takes a calling!

What is a "vocation"? The dictionary explains: "A strong feeling of suitability for a particular career or occupation; an inclination, as if in response to a calling."[4]

I sometimes wonder if I had the vocation to be a doctor, and especially to be an oncologist. I already thought I did not, since I have abandoned my profession when I moved to Quebec. Of course, I have attempt-

---

3 http://www.cqai.com.br
4 http://oxforddictionaries.com and http://www.thefreedictionary.com.

ed to pursue it here, but I did not manage to get the license for practicing Medicine, and I had a good reason for moving to Canada: I found my happiness with my Quebecer, as you all know, "*qui prend mari, prend pays.*"[5] *Et voilà!*

Anyway, working as a medical oncologist for twenty years has allowed me to acquire a broad enough experience. I saw the disease in the most diverse range of stages, affecting people from different regions, from all social classes, with huge differences in the level of information. I followed cases of victory and cases of failure. It is not easy, and we only realize its magnitude when we go completely out of the "scenario."

Doctors are so busy studying, evaluating and treating their patients, that they cannot indulge in the luxury of being emotional. Indeed, they are often accused of indifference, because they are very concise during consultations and patient follow-up, showing an apparent insensitivity. This is quite normal, and involuntary; it is a defense, to keep their emotional integrity. In my opinion, it is the correct attitude. Doctors must treat many patients, and they must keep the reason, the intellect, in the best possible con-

---

5 From French: "Whoever takes a husband, takes a country."

ditions to make important decisions on behalf of their patients.

I have accomplished this ritual during my time as an oncologist, with the exception of the last two years, after I lost my sister to cancer. I remember once, after receiving a woman patient in consultation with her own sister, I burst into tears, as if they were my sister and myself who had just left my office. And the patient's sister found me in this condition when she returned to my office, to ask additional questions. I did not have time to hide my grief, and I had to tell her what was happening, or she would think her sister was dying.

I was no longer the same person; and this helped me to accept the choice of giving up my profession, when I decided to stay in Quebec.

Finally, this whole context left me important scars. I congratulate the doctors who have experienced similar situations and kept control of their emotional side. It is admirable! And it must be so. Otherwise, we lose the necessary skills for being a doctor.

It seems to me that once a doctor, always a doctor — exactly like the priests. I do not misrepresent the saying completely, because here I am, writing about this subject, which still remains in my thoughts.

As we try to better understand the oncologist, this strange character, we could say the madness begins with their interest in science. To study the effects of chemotherapy, for example, we must study the innermost vital mechanisms of the cells of our body, because it is where the drugs will act. It is fascinating! When we study the pharmacological basis for the mechanism of action in cancer treatment, we become optimistic about the possibility of healing. The struggle, which takes place in the deep structure of the cell, the action of chemotherapeutic molecules to trap the cell in a moment, or a target point, in order to destroy it — this whole stuff is very interesting for someone who has an inclination for science and for the mysteries of life. It motivates even more doctors who chose to be oncologists; and they are tempted to continue the fight against death, touching vital points... as paradoxical as it may sound.

In oncology, there is also another factor that keeps doctors' hopes always alive: This is one of the specializations in which the sharing of knowledge is done more intensely. Countless are the scientific and professional meetings carried out locally, regionally, internationally, all over the world, with the exchange of results, including rigorous statistical studies. In this way, treatment protocols spread globally, and the oncologists feel themselves immersed in a network where they can learn, and, at the same time, give their own contribution, being updated continuously.

### The role of pharmaceutical companies

The time has come to mention the role played by pharmaceutical companies. We know they have a high economic interest at stake; but we must consider their importance in the development and progress of cancer treatment, because these companies infiltrate in the most remote and hidden corners of the planet with their representatives, bringing their products to the attention of doctors. This interest in sales ends up being very useful for the standardization of oncologic approaches, when combined with access to networks of treatment protocols, and criteria for the use of drugs in an increasingly stringent cancer treatment. This is also a good way to study new treatment protocols, because there are more patients being evaluated, and, consequently, more reliable results.

Nevertheless, caution is advised; in their judgment, physicians must rest assured of always making the right choices, and the right choice for doctors is to take care of their patients' health, not to serve economic interests. We must always rely on studies that have shown ample efficacy. In the case of experimental studies, it is essential to follow the most stringent scientific criteria. We cannot ignore a treatment recognized as successful in order to try new approaches, without a clear evidence of the need to change.

### The famous risk-benefit ratio

Moreover, the judgment ability must always be very sharp in this profession. Another situation requiring this skill is the search for a better solution of conflicts, when several morbidity circumstances are considered.

Oncologists should be able to analyze the risk-benefit ratio of a treatment accurately. In other words, they must be aware of a treatment that becomes more dangerous than the disease itself. Doctors must face some very complex situations; for example, when we know that the treatment must be aggressive to achieve the cure, to the point of putting the patients' lives at risk. In some cases, it is necessary to take this risk, but, of course, we must notify the patients and their families of these conditions, to obtain their permission to do so.

Accurate judgment is also required in

situations on the other extremity, for example, to decide when to stop the treatment when it becomes counterproductive. When the cure is not possible, the goal of the treatment must be to favor a better quality of life, associated with a longer survival; there is a time when the treatment becomes useless, only leading to more suffering.

There are many different conditions needing different kinds of treatment. The disease may have a chronic behavior, for example. And it may be treated like many other conditions that will not be cured, but do not threaten life immediately, requiring a chronic treatment as well.

The judgment of physicians is always important; we must allow them to work in the best possible conditions, in order to maximize the possibility of the best decision-making, resulting in better outcomes.

### Working together

In this context of "the best possible" and "the best decisions," team working is a good option for the exchange of opinions among colleagues, which can be done daily; everyone benefits. If a doctor reaches a dead-end when dealing with a complicated case, a brief meeting with other doctors can be held, in a conference room, to discuss how to conduct the case, while the patient is waiting in the doctor's office. This procedure prevents unnecessary delays in the decision-making, and, consequently, in the treatment.

This situation is also reassuring for patients, because they know there are surrogates who are aware of their case, ready to replace their doctor in case of their absence. It is reassuring for doctors as well, to know that another oncologist of their own team is ready to take care of their patients, in case of impediment.

### The infamous cost-benefit ratio

Nowadays, we hear a lot about the cost-benefit ratio of treatments. I do not think this is an analysis that should occupy the mind of the physician, and this comes as a warning. I do not see its purpose for the well-being of the patient, and this criterion does not please me.

I know this is a very controversial subject; I think it is a reflection of the evolution of civilization, which is still passing through transformations, and is, at present, chaotic. We are losing parameters and criteria. The hierarchy of values is changing; and is still completely anarchic and disturbed. I hope it will achieve balance one day. It is essential to consider the patient as the main priority of the physician; emphasizing it is never too much.

### The omnipotence: domination x submission

With all these challenges and all the qualifications needed to be a good doctor, we understand that pride comes to the list. This is normal, even necessary to play such a demanding role. We also understand that this pride can sometimes overflow; we should always be careful to avoid feeling all powerful, because we are very far from this condition. In reality, limitless power does not exist in this perishable universe. It would be too ridiculous to act as if we had it.

Sometimes, patients manifest an exaggerated reverence towards their doctors, in a real play of domination versus submission. It happened more often in the past. Today, the doctor-patient relationship has changed a lot, thanks to easier access to information for everyone, including patients, and this level of communication is increasingly present in decision-making. But we must not exaggerate; patients do not have the required knowledge and training to decide about their treatment. Even when patients are doctors, their emotional state is not always stable enough to be able to make decisions about their own illness.

### A testimony

Finally, what is the purpose of these thoughts about the oncologist? I still have lots of questions. Why did I have a kind of "calling" to write about this theme? Could my book help others on their journey? Yes. I think so.

Sharing our experiences is very important, it helps us improve, and it makes us move forward. I witnessed a lot of suffering; and I saw many examples of courage and solidarity — the human being is always surprising, we are not a lost cause at all. I saw the efforts of physicians trying to overcome difficulties, always in search of the best results. I have also seen the evolution of treatments over time.

Sometimes, I feel guilty for leaving my people behind, my poor patients, but this feeling fades away when I remember that I dedicated to them most part of my life, the best of my youth. Now, I want to leave a message of encouragement, an incitement to "life," through the oncologist I once was.

I think there is still a long way to go, a lot of research to be done. But I am optimistic; great strides have been made, I am a witness. We are much more hopeful today than when I started in the profession.

I have some suggestions — supplications, rather — for the oncologists:

— Always keep an attitude of investigation, sharp in all senses; always ask yourself if you are following the right path;

— It would be desirable to conduct more research in cancer treatment and to target different points of action; I think we could have another approach, in terms of cell division, as I mentioned in Chapter 2;

— Plan your work shift and your time of rest, and if you feel tired, discouraged, take your time to recharge the batteries; but do not let your colleagues alone in the battle; especially, do not let your patients without consolation. Please, do not give up!

## 5. Conclusion

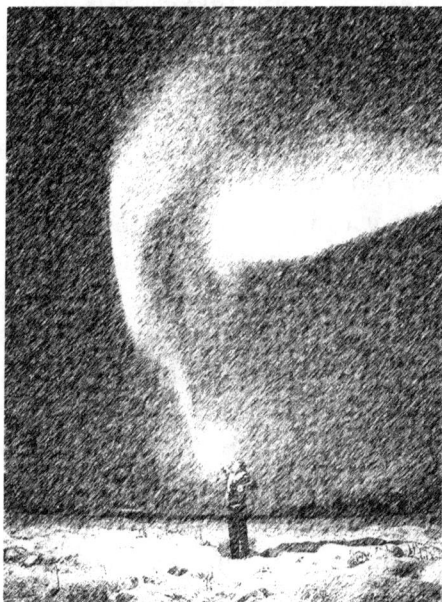

In order to practice our ability to get perplexed, I will now give you some surprising information, which is not often discussed with the general public. Some kinds of cancer come into spontaneous regression! Yes, it is possible! It gives us the shivers, doesn't it?

The classic example is a tumor that may affect young children, the disease being present at birth — the neuroblastoma. It does not happen in all cases of neuroblastoma, of course, but it happens. Oncologists know this phenomenon, although there are some who have never seen it in their daily practice.

I have seen several cases of neuroblastoma, in all stages, because I worked for a long time in the field of oncology and in the reference center of a densely populated area. And yes, I have seen cases of spontaneous complete remission.

In my opinion, it reinforces my proposal for a new approach in the cancer treatment: To start trying to make the cancer cell return to a normal pace of multiplication, instead of simply destroying it, as I said in the Chapter 2. We should not always think in terms of destruction. We must change this standard. We have to make radical changes!

Sometimes, I feel as if we were prisoners in a game, ignoring its most basic rules. But I hope we will find this trap that catches us, and we will get rid of it. Everything that seems mysterious or surrounded by mysticism, the maze that makes us turn in circles, in random trial and error, yes, it will be clarified someday. For now, it is just a Belief... with a capital B!

I have no definitive conclusions to offer

for the moment. Reflection is required when it comes to the observation of facts. We must always ask questions...

Humanity is extraordinary! In a perspective view, I always arrive to this amazing thought. We live in an inhospitable, cruel universe. And we are so good, so innocent — I would say naive — that we are able to find nature beautiful, this nature based entirely on pain, even in its most ordinary occurrences. We brutally root out a plant — a gesture considered harmless — and thank nature for giving it to us as food. In reality, we should not need to be thankful, because nature will take it back, one day.

I hope my words are not too hard...

I am just trying to understand how our environment works. It seems to me that every event happening in this universe is an attempt to make life possible. However, life depends on the other's death — this is not what I would call "perfection." Despite this mess, we have a kind of ancestral instinct, I would dare say, an ancestral memory of survival; we are always trying to recover, an impulse leading us to progress. Whatever it is, something wrong must have happened to the universe that it ended up in such imperfection. There must be something wider out there that what we cannot fathom for now...

In another scale, it could be something

similar to the agent that damages the cell and triggers its desperate multiplication, despite the harmful effects caused to other tissues and even leading to the loss of the whole organism. I get more and more convinced that the behavior of the cancer cell is a desperate attempt to survive after an injury caused by a harmful agent, like radiation, just to mention one. The damage it causes is interpreted as a lethal danger, and the cell starts to act according to an almost invincible mechanism of multiplication, in order to keep itself alive. But it is chaotic, and it leads to disproportionate consequences. It is the power of life acting on a system that is in error — a "basic" error.

Please, at this moment, let us take a break to think about what I have just said.

At a universal level, something drastically wrong really must have happened to life in order to explain all this chaotic condition, not perfect at all. It is very tempting to believe in a damaging agent affecting the universe, and it could be something some religions call "original sin." Obviously, I do not believe in traditional narratives literally; they are full of allegories, but probably as a result of inspired philosophical thoughts.

What did in fact happen? I do not know. We are too insignificant to realize how, and why. But the result is clear for everyone to see: every single unit in this universe is trying to survive and cannot escape death.

Let us think together about how to overcome death... There should be a key to open this immense closed door! All of us, in communion, will find the way to life without death. It sounds like religious reasoning... Maybe religion and science are closer than we think.

Many philosophers tried to explain the mystery of life, and their writings are usually too complicated to understand. It is not surprising. How to establish a rationale of something we do not know entirely?

Now, I want to change the tone. Throughout this book I tried to manage the words to avoid falling into the futility of sentimentality. But now I want to speak softly. The time has come to write about humanity and human nature, about all of us, with a little tenderness.

As we become older, we gain a few skills, like the ability of better analyzing our situation, although limited by our own conditioning. Despite all limitations, I realize that humanity is making a "superhuman" effort — if we may say so. And it makes me believe the human being is so much more than we can imagine! We try to overcome our own instincts; we are able to organize ourselves and to process our misfortunes.

Humanity is walking against the current. It is impossible to be skeptical! I hope we will continue our evolution in an intelligent way, despite all the stupidity humans are still capable of.

Cancer is a phenomenon that triggers a burst of union among humans. In a way, it highlights our sensitivity side, our empathy towards our neighbor. The sense of urgency and solidarity is present at all levels.

Throughout my years of practice, I witnessed many acts of indulgence, kindness and generosity. Even in the tortuous bureaucratic ways of public health systems, we can detect the presence of compassion in the background. Not to mention the countless non-profit organizations helping people affected by the disease and its consequences, and also many gestures of solidarity among the population, individually or through associations and public campaigns.

This human behavior is a sign of LIFE. We are not made to die so abruptly; there is something that does not seem to be consistent with the essence of our existence. Let us make more efforts together... May the motto of the oncologist, "For a longer survival and better quality of life," become unanimity.

May the good "Aurora Polaris" show up in all latitudes, in all its fullness and magnitude...

## Aurora Borealis

*This is what I see*
*Only a beautiful rainbow*
*Ephemeral*
*A seducing light spectrum*
*Formed by some circumstances*
*Produced at random, like me*
*In my genetic circumstances*
*Adrift in an ocean*
*Where I am decomposing*
*In the events*
*Even in the last moment*
*When I die*
*Ephemeral*
*I can choose the purple rose*
*As my favorite color*
*While blue is the most loved one*
*But nothing changes*
*Not even my weight*
*I need to see*
*One day*
*An aurora borealis*
*Illuminating the endless night*
*Sweeping in flames*
*The cruel random sky*